The 5:2 Diet
RECIPES

Easy, Tasty, Calorie-counted Dishes
to Make Your Fasting Days Delicious!

James Drummond

The 5:2 Diet
RECIPES

Eat Whatever You Want 5 Days a Week!

Easy, Tasty, Calorie-counted Dishes
to Make Your Fasting Days Delicious!

Discover the revolutionary new eating plan that everyone is talking about!

This breakthrough technique allows you to activate your "skinny gene" and enjoy consistent weight loss, increase your health and well-being and live a longer and healthier life! All in just 2 days a week!

* *Lose weight easily and quickly without depriving yourself every single day.*

* *"Diet" just 2 days a week – eat as normal the other 5 days!*

* *Choose from an array of simple, tasty low-calorie recipes to make your Fast days delicious!*

* *100, 200 and 300 calorie snacks, breakfasts, lunches and dinners to keep you fuller, longer.*

A Kyle Craig Publication

www.kyle-craig.com

First published in 2013 by Kyle Craig Publishing

Text & illustration copyright © Kyle Craig Publishing

ISBN 978-1-908707-22-2

Disclaimer

The information and advice contained in this book is intended as a general guide. The author or publisher shall not be liable for any loss or damage allegedly arising from any information or suggestion in this book. Always consult your doctor before embarking on any diet or change of eating habits.

Eat Whatever You Want 5 Days a Week!

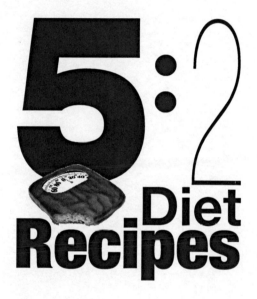

5:2 Diet Recipes

Easy, Tasty, Calorie-counted Dishes to Make Your Fasting Days Delicious!

James Drummond

Contents

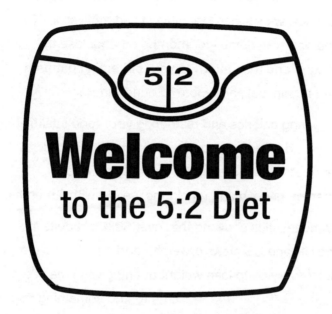

Welcome
to the 5:2 Diet

Bored of dieting?

Do you manage to stick to each new weight-loss regime for a few weeks then lose interest and motivation? Or you deprive yourself for months on end, lose the weight, and then return to your old eating patterns and regain it all, and more? Sound familiar?

Counting calories and restricting your food intake day in, day out can soon become tedious — "diet fatigue" kicks in — and the majority of us lose interest, give up and regain the weight within months.

With statistics showing that over 60% of adults in the UK and US are overweight, and 1 in 3 of us are actively trying to lose weight at any given time, it's time to find something that really works, and is sustainable in the long term.

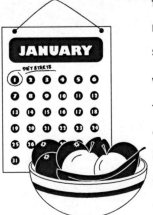

We all want to look better, feel better, have more energy and improve our health and vitality. But we don't want to have to give up the foods we love.

Imagine a diet where you could eat whatever you wanted, pretty much most of the time. No foods would be out of bounds, you wouldn't have to count calories every day, or avoid certain food groups. But you could still lose weight, feel better and live longer. Wouldn't that be great?

Scientists have known since the 1930s that one of the best ways to lose weight and extend life is to eat a nutritionally rich but calorie-restricted diet. Tests have shown that mice on such a diet live up to 40 per cent longer than normal mice. The trouble is, not many of us can realistically live on a severely calorie-restricted diet for our whole lives.

One popular method of restricting calories is called *Intermittent Fasting*, and scientists have uncovered evidence that short periods of fasting, if properly controlled, could achieve a number of health benefits, as well as result in significant weight loss.

A recent BBC documentary saw Dr. Michael J. Mosley investigate the practice of calorie restriction and the benefits of fasting on our health and well-being.

Rather than the Intermittent Fasting, or 'fasting every other day' practiced by some, Mosley decided to adopt a more manageable "5-2 Diet", where a typical week is made up of 5 days of normal eating and 2 days of "fasting". On the "fast" days, women are allowed to eat a total of 500 calories (men 600 calories) per day.

Starting out at 13½ st, Mosley decided to embark on a 6 week trial to monitor the impact of this 5:2 diet plan.

Six weeks later, the results were impressive. He had lost well over a stone, and 25% of his body fat. His blood glucose levels, which had been borderline diabetic, were normal and his cholesterol levels, previously high enough to necessitate medication, were also down in the healthy range. He also dropped from the "overweight" category according to BMI and into the healthy weight category.

But the big news was that by fasting 2 days a week his blood glucose levels fell, so he was at a much lower risk of developing diabetes. His cholesterol levels fell too, which reduced his risk of heart disease. Mosley concluded that fasting was definitely a way to help people reduce their weight, manage their health and significantly reduce their risk of developing the big killers in the West — heart disease and diabetes.

So how does the 5:2 diet work, and how can you incorporate this easily into your own life?
Read on......

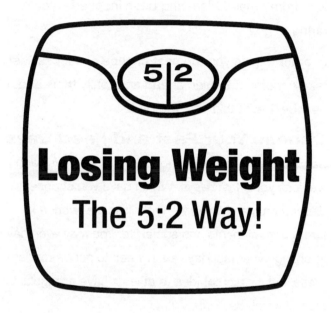

So, you're all set to get cracking on the 5:2 – you've bought the books and learned all about the health benefits, you've read the amazing stories of weight-loss from other 5:2'ers and been inspired – you're raring to go !

In order to give you the best chance of success, let's take a moment to plan ahead and really think about how best to fit this into your life.

Choose Your Fast and Feed Days

So you need to choose 2 nonconsecutive days each week as your "fast" days. Which days you choose will depend on many factors — your lifestyle, work and family commitments and social life. You may even have to change your fast days each week to accommodate these, but it's a great idea to at least have a "regular" plan of which days you will fast.

I personally go for Monday's and Wednesdays, and this is a popular choice for most 5:2 'ers. After a weekend of eating and drinking, I'm almost pleased to be eating less on a Monday, and I find that this is by far my easiest fast day.

Wednesdays also work for me as it's still early in the week and I can try to schedule any social outings

— meals or drinks with friends — for the Thursday, Friday or weekend. If something comes up on a Wednesday that can't be moved, I can still bump my fast day along to Thursday and it still doesn't impact on my weekend fun!

Think about which days will work best for you, and plan accordingly. And that includes food and grocery shopping, which we'll look at next.

Food

One of the happy side effects of fasting a couple of days a week, is that your grocery bills will become trimmer too! You're eating less, so you should be spending less. Result! During the first week or two of being on the 5:2, I made the mistake of shopping as normal — doing one large "shop" for the week and having a fridge full of food.

I found that not only was it harder to stick to my fast days when I was presented with a fridge full of lovely food each time I opened the door, I also ended up throwing so much away as I was simply eating less, and fresh foods were expiring before I could use them.

17

Now I plan my week carefully, look at what I will eat for each fast and feed day and shop accordingly. I live alone, so this is pretty easy, but those of you with families may find that it's simply a case of tweaking your usual dishes and making less of something when you're on your fast day.

I tend to shop on a Friday for my Fri/Sat/Sunday and "fast" Monday meals, then again on a Tuesday for my Tuesday, "fast" Wednesday and Thursday meals.

While this may not be ideal for those of you with busy jobs and lives, it's good to find what works best for you and through trial and error you'll arrive at a way of food planning and shopping that works for you and your family.

Fast Days

On your Fast days, the plan is to consume **500** *for women and* **600** *calories for men.*

Because there have been few human trials of the 5:2 diet, no one is certain whether it is better to eat those calories in one meal or to spread them out through the day.

Dr Michael Mosley went for a split: 300 calories for breakfast and 300 for supper. Because I've never been much of a breakfast person — I tend to feel quite squeamish for the first couple of hours at least — eating in the morning isn't important to me. So I try to use 200 calories at lunchtime, or as late as I can stand — sometimes as late as 2 or 2.30pm if I can hold out that long. Then I have the remainder in the evening for a tasty meal. The lunch or snack satisfies my daytime hunger pangs, but saving the bulk of my calories for my evening meal means that I also have something tasty to look forward to at the end of the day.

Some people who have incredibly busy jobs may find it relatively easy to get through the whole day on just liquids and save their calories for their evening meal. Find whatever works for you.

In the next section of the book are a ton of delicious and nutritious recipes to help you plan your meals. Because each of us will choose to spread our calorie allowance differently, these recipes have been organised by calorie amount — this way you can mix and match depending on your hunger levels and what sort of sized dish you wish to eat and when.

You'll notice that these dishes are based on lots of fresh and nutritious ingredients, and that's the real key to this whole 5:2 thing. Sure, you could in theory "spend" your entire daily calorie allowance on a Mars bar and 2 glasses of wine and still be technically sticking to the rules, but your body would soon show its disapproval! Making sure your body has all the essential nutrients and goodness to function is so important, plus you'll feel more energised, less lethargic and fuller longer if you choose the best possible fuel for your body.

While the first few fast days may prove difficult — you may struggle to control the hunger pangs and feel tired or irritable — many 5:2 dieters report increase feelings of energy and alertness once they adjust to the 5:2 plan.

Feed Days

On your Feed days, you're allowed to eat whatever you want, and that is one of the main attractions to the 5:2 plan! However, if you use this as an excuse to gorge yourself on huge amounts of junk food and cakes, and consume thousands of extra calories that you wouldn't usually, then it will come as no surprise that you won't lose weight and may even gain some. This is a diet, not a miracle cure for obesity!

Research by US Scientist Dr Krista Varady of the University of Chicago showed that a test group following an alternate day fasting regime actually didn't consume a whole lot more on their Feed days than they usually would – perhaps 110% of their usual calorie intake. Many 5:2 'ers reported that their appetites actually decreased overall, and they were less hungry the day after a fast day than they would be usually, so they naturally ate less even on a feed day.

You would imagine that you would awake ravenous after a fast day — after all you have probably spent most of the previous day dreaming of all the delicious foods that you can't wait to eat — but strangely that it not the case for many of us.

I know that I am usually not hungry until at least lunchtime the day after a fast day, so I happily skip breakfast and then enjoy whatever I feel like for lunch and dinner.

It seems that by fasting and pressing "pause" on the constant food assault on our bodies, we help "reset" our hunger buttons and become more in tune with our true hunger. By feeling and acknowledging hunger, but failing to respond to it and letting it pass on our fast days, we are actually learning to control our appetites and really listen to our bodies.

Like a naughty toddler constantly acting out to get our attention, hunger is something that we must learn to control and not immediately react to, stuffing it with treats and snacks to silence it!

Adding In An Extra Day; Alternate Day Fasting

The basis of much of the research to date has been on Alternate Day Fasting — or fasting every other day. It was this initial plan that led to Mosley's idea for a less severe version, the 5:2. However, those with a large amount of weight to lose, or who want to really kick-start their 5:2 life, may decide to try adding a third fast day in.

If you're currently fasting Mondays and Wednesdays, then Friday seems like the obvious 3rd day. For me personally, I like to look forward to a glass of wine and a nice meal on a Friday evening, so I go for a 2½ day fast plan.

I fast as usual Monday and Wednesday, then on Thursday, my "feed" day, I have my meal at 7pm and that is the last thing I eat. I then fast until 7pm Friday, but am free to enjoy my Friday evening as I wish. This works well for me as I get the best of both worlds — an extra day but with little impact on my weekend and social life.

Stay Hydrated

Even when we're not on any sort of diet plan, it's important to stay hydrated, and the reality is that many of us do not drink enough water in a typical day. Too often, we mistake hunger for thirst and reach for snacks when in fact a large glass of water is sufficient to calm our "hunger" and help us regain our focus. Water is your friend — not only will keeping hydrated help you stay alert and full of energy, it will help you feel "full" and distract you from any fast day hunger pangs.

Whether you prefer to buy bottled water, or like to use your own filtered water, keep several bottles wherever you may need them — in the car, on your desk, chilling in the fridge.

Each morning I take a large sports bottle with water to my desk, and have 3 more in the fridge — and by the end of each day all 4 have gone and I wash and refill them ready for the next day. On fast days, when hunger threatens to get the better of me, I take a drink of water, or make some tea, and the hunger quickly passes.

Caffeinated Drinks

One common myth is that caffeine causes dehydration, when in fact, up to 6 cups of coffee a day does not increase diuresis any more than plain water. So beverages containing caffeine can make up at least part of your daily fluid intake.

Many people on the 5:2 diet report a significant increase in energy as a result of fasting, and this, combined with extra caffeine intake, could result in sleeping issues. If this sounds like you, or you are particularly sensitive to caffeine anyway, perhaps limit your caffeine intake, especially later in the day.

Alcohol

Many of us look forward to a relaxing glass of wine in the evenings, to help unwind after a busy day. But can we continue this while on the 5:2 plan?

On a fasting day, the simple answer is: probably not. Sure, you could use a chunk of your valuable 5/600

calorie allocation on booze, but wouldn't you rather
have a decent meal instead? Plus, drinking on such a
low calorie intake could leave you feeling woozy, give
you a crazy headache, and make you feel even worse
the next day. Is it really so difficult to abstain for 2
days out of each week?

On your feed days, whether you drink or not will be
up to you and how it makes you feel. I was used
to having a couple of glasses of red wine most
evenings, but now find that if I have even a couple
of glasses of wine on the feed night before a fast day,
I wake up feeling slightly hungover and craving carbs
and comfort food.

It makes my fast day 100 times more difficult than
usual, so now I choose not to drink on a Sunday or
Tuesday evening, before each fast day. And since
I don't drink on a fast day either, this actually means
that I now don't alcohol drink Sunday-Wednesday
but can do what I like Thursdays, Fridays and
Saturdays. So another great side effect of embarking
on the 5:2 plan is that I have managed to cut down
on my mid week wine habit, and I feel hugely better
for this too.

Exercising While on The 5:2 Diet

The main reason for weight gain, and the increase in body fat as we age is a decrease in our metabolism. Research has shown that most people's metabolisms decrease 0.5% percent per year after the age of 25.

The three main factors that slow down a person's metabolism are:

* *Decrease in muscle mass*

* *Change in hormone levels*

* *Decreased caloric need of internal organs.*

All three of these factors can be controlled by making lifestyle changes. The one that is the most controllable is the decrease in muscle mass.

Basically, we lose muscle cells as we age. When younger muscle cells get damaged, they're quickly repaired. That's not the case with older muscles, according to UCLA researcher and geriatrician Jonathan Wanagat. He says we don't know why muscles literally shrink as we age. But there are a number of theories.

"I think one of the ones that have become increasingly interesting and popular is the idea that the stem cells

*in the muscle are not able to respond to damage or to
aging the way they did when we were younger,"* says
Wanagat. And if damaged muscle cells aren't repaired,
they sort of whittle away and die, he says. Decreases
in growth hormone, testosterone and estrogen levels
may also account for the loss of muscle fibre and the
inability of tissue to replenish itself.

In addition, the muscle cells we're left with are sort
of worn out, according to Wanagat. *"If you think of
muscles as being the energy powerhouse of our body,
that's where most of our calories are burned. And
when we talk about metabolism, what we're really
talking about is how efficiently those powerhouse cells
— the muscle cells of our body — burn the energy
we bring in."*

Energy is delivered to the body in the form of calories.
And if you keep your caloric intake exactly the same
as you get older, those unburned calories end up as
fat.

The best way to build muscle is through strength
training — toning and building muscles using
equipment like handheld weights, elastic bands,

or the machines and weight training equipment found in your local gym.

Strength Training (also called Resistance Training) is based on working specific muscles or muscle groups to "failure" (the point at which you can't do another repetition) in order to increase their mass and strength.

As well as doing some strength or resistance training, it's also important to do some cardiovascular activity such as walking, biking, running or swimming, as this improves your heart function by helping it pump more efficiently.

On your fast days you may find that strength training is fine, but any increase in your aerobic activity can lead to increased hunger and tiredness. You can exercise as normal on your feed days — so perhaps mix things up by dedicating fast days to either no workouts, or light strength training only, and save your running or swimming for a feed day.

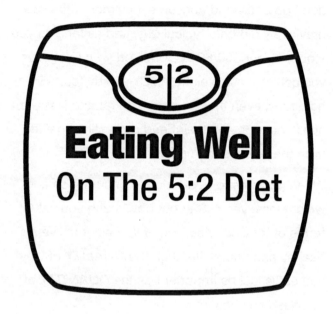

5|2

Eating Well
On The 5:2 Diet

One of the things that most attracts people to the 5:2 diet is the promise that you can eat *WHATEVER YOU LIKE* on your Feed days and, as long as you don't go crazy and consume way more than you previously did on a typical day, and as long as you stock to your 500/600 calories on your Fast days, you can still lose weight. As Dr Varady found in her study, even those eating high fat and less than healthy options on their Feed days still benefited from the key health improvements of ADF.

When it comes to total calorie consumption and weight loss, yes it IS about how much you eat in terms of total calories…but if you want to live a healthy and happy life, then the *QUALITY* of what you eat is just as important as the *QUANTITY* of calories you consume.

The tests on ADF so far have only been run over relatively short periods of time, and cannot possibly show the impact any sort of diet or eating regime will have on the human body for the long term. One thing we do know, however, is that we and our bodies function better, and receive greater health benefits, when we eat well. Fruit and vegetables, whole grains, clean, lean and nutritious foods that provide the fuel we need for our bodies to thrive.

So it's important to think carefully about what we choose to eat on both our Feed and Fast days. Now this is not a sneaky attempt to contradict the initial claim that you can still eat exactly what you like 5 days a week. On the contrary — it's more about paying attention to what you eat, on your Feed days but even more so on your Fast days.

My view is that if I'm only allowed 600 calories today, then I want to make sure I "spend" those on the tastiest, most filling and satisfying meals and snacks that I can. I don't want to feel like I'm on a diet or depriving myself or even consciously counting calories. I just want to live, and eat according to the plan while I'm at it.

If there is any hope for us to make 5:2 a way of life, a way of keeping the natural weight gain of middle-age at bay, and enjoy all the associated health benefits of fasting, then we need to find an eating plan that is easy, delicious, nutritious and filling.

Here follows a selection of truly delicious recipes that all have one great thing in common — they are nutritious and full of good, healthy ingredients. And they happen to be low enough in calories to be incorporated into a 5:2 Fast day.

Some of them you may love so much you even make them on a Feed day too! Once you've tried enough of these, you'll no doubt have a handful of favourites that you return to on each Fast day — making it even easier to plan your week, your grocery shopping and your family meals.

No doubt you will also create some recipes of your own, based on your favourite foods, and I daresay some of us may even sneak the odd ready-meal into the mix. (While many ready meals may boast a low calorie content, beware that they may be high in sugar and salt to make up for this, so look carefully at the label to see what is really in there, and try to use these sparingly.)

Life is busy and time is short, so find what works best for you and stick with it!

RECIPES

Breakfasts
Under 100 Calories

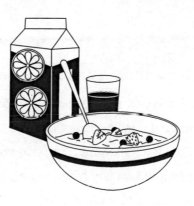

Vanilla and Banana Smoothie

(½ Cup Banana, ¼ Vanilla Yoghurt and Ice)

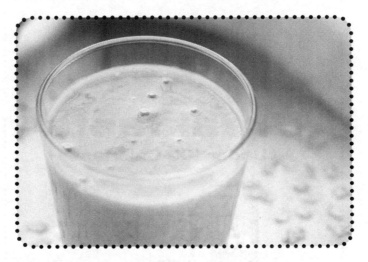

The ice is the key to this delicious smoothie —
it transforms the vanilla, banana, and calcium-rich
yoghurt into a thicker, more filling, ice creamy
substance that will satisfy a serious sweet tooth.
Add all ingredients to a blender and whizz for
1 minute.

½ Cup Puffed Rice with Skimmed Milk and a Handful of Berries

A handful of antioxidant-rich berries and a splash of
calcium filled, low-fat skimmed milk, added to half a
cup of cereal is nutritionally sound way to start your day.

1 Grapefruit with 1 tsp Sugar

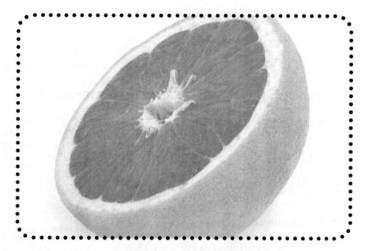

Eating a grapefruit with a sprinkling of sugar is a diet snack that dates back years. As well as containing high levels of vitamin C, grapefruit contains a naturally occurring chemical that lowers insulin levels, reducing cravings and increasing the body's ability to burn fat.

¼ Cup of Muesli with Skimmed Milk

Granola or muesli is another great way to start your day. Tho oombination of grains, oats and bran that granola contains will provide your body with a steady source of energy, as well as B vitamins and fibre.

Meanwhile, the calcium-rich skimmed milk will contribute to a fuller, more satisfied feeling that will last through the day.

1 Plain Bagel with Low-Fat Spread

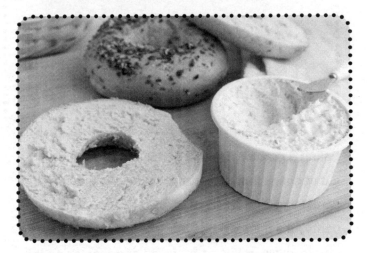

Check the calorie content of your usual bagel brand – if you're lucky, or by scooping out the filling or going for half a bagel, you can enjoy this for under 100 calories. If you go for the wholemeal option, a bagel will provide you with a good source of complex carbohydrates and energy-boosting B vitamins.

1 Poached Egg and 1 tsp Light Hollandaise Sauce

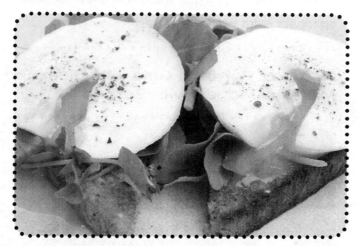

Eggs are super filling, because they're packed with protein, essential Omega 3 fats, selenium and other vitamins and minerals, making them a nutritious snack. Poaching is better than frying, because, as it's cooked in water, the egg retains less of the fat used in the cooking process.

1 Toasted Crumpet with Thin Slice of Cheese

Crumpets are a great, low-cal way of getting your carbs fix, but without blowing the calories. Calcium-rich foods, like cheese, are good for providing a feeling of fullness, so grill yours with a low-fat slice on top for extra yum.

⅓ Cup of Porridge Oats with Skimmed Milk and Topped with Berries

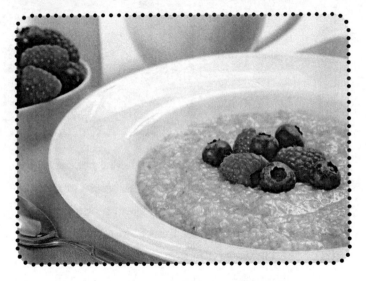

Oats are vitamin-rich, high in dissolvable fibre, protein and minerals, and provide your body with slow-release energy to keep you going without feeling hungry. Coupled with skimmed milk and a handful of antioxidant-rich berries? You've got all the main food groups covered in one.

Boiled Egg and Soldiers
(1 Runny Egg with ½ Slice Bread)

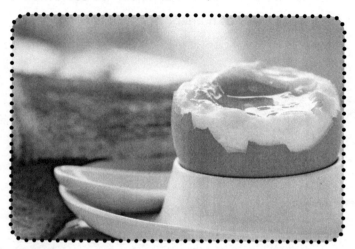

Go back to your childhood, with a delicious breakfast of dippy egg and soldiers! Eggs are filling because they are high in protein and other nutrients, while wholemeal bread is a rich source of complex carbohydrates.

Strawberry, Peanut Butter and Skimmed Milk Smoothie
(8 Strawberries, 1 tsp Peanut Butter, ½ Skimmed Milk with Ice)

This skimmed milkshake is every bit as delicious as it sounds — and filling, too. Blend eight strawberries

41

together with half a glass of skimmed milk, a tsp of peanut butter and a handful of ice for a tasty meal in a glass that's as nutrient-rich as it is filling.

100 Calories
Snacks & Treats

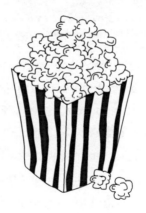

2 Small Falafels

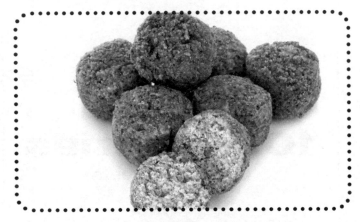

Like most other pulses, chickpeas are a cheap way to pack a lot of different nutrients into your diet for relatively few calories: fibre, complex carbohydrates, protein, iron, vitamins B6, C and K. Falafels are a particularly delicious way to enjoy them, especially when you consider the metabolism-boosting benefits of the spices they contain. Go for grilled falafels to keep the calorie count to a minimum.

Green Leaf Salad with Cider Vinegar Dressing, Cucumber, Pepper, Onion and Plum Tomatoes

You can eat an awful lot of salad without using up too many calories, which makes it a great Fast day

option. The combination of fibre and different
vitamins and minerals makes it highly nutritious,
while the cider vinegar dressing adds a metabolism-
boosting kick.

Hummus and Mini Wholewheat Pitta

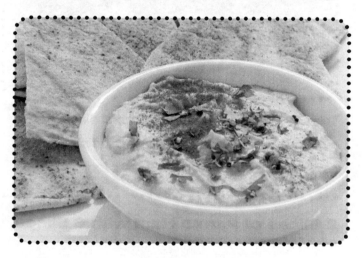

Choose low fat hummus and wholemeal pitta bread,
and this is a very good snack or mini meal indeed.
The chickpeas and wholegrains combined provide
just the right combination of fibre, protein, complex
carbohydrates and metabolism-boosting vitamins
and minerals you need to keep you going until your
next meal.

Tomato, Feta and Olive Salad

(1 Tom/1 tbsp Feta/5 Olives)

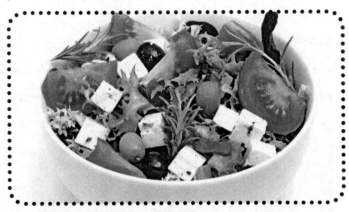

This Greek delicacy combines several different nutritional elements to create a snack dish that is as filling as it is beneficial. And tasty too!

2 Slices of Parma Ham with 6 Slices of Melon

Yes, you read this correctly — *SIX* slices of melon! Good old melon. It's always a great option for a diet snack, and is even tastier when teamed with a few super thin slices of Parma ham. This delicious Italian dish works particularly well because it combines the high water, fibre and vitamin content of the melon with the protein of the ham.

2 Small Bruschetta Toast with Tomato Salsa

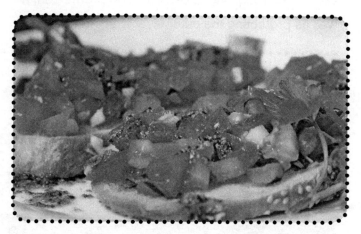

Toast 2 slices of ciabatta bread, then whip up some tomato salsa (diced tomatoes with chopped onions and coriander), and you've got a snack that will keep you satisfied without tipping your calorie count over the edge.

1 Serving of Tomato Soup

Tomato soup is a great low calorie snack, and tasty too! Tomatoes are high in vitamin C, which helps support a healthy immune system, as well as fibre. Red vegetables, like tomatoes, also contain a naturally-occurring plant chemical called lycopene

— a powerful antioxidant that encourages skin elasticity through increased collagen production, as well as protecting the outer layer from sun damage.

8 King Prawns with a Sweet Chilli Dipping Sauce

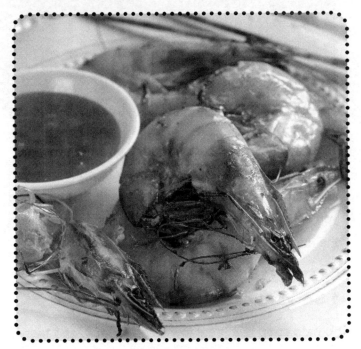

Sizzle the prawns in a non-stick pan then dip in a small amount of delicious sweet chilli sauce for a super tasty and nutritious snack!

1 tsp Cream Cheese on 1 Ryvita with a Tomato

It might not seem like much, but the nutrient-packed blend of cream cheese (full of calcium and protein), Ryvita (fibre and B vitamins) and tomatoes (vitamin C and collagen-boosting lycopene) is more than enough to keep hunger pangs at bay on a Fast day.

1 Small Baked Potato

A small baked jacket potato is an excellent energy-rich and diet-friendly snack. Just make sure it's not dripping in butter or toppings, and that you eat the skin, too — it's rich in B vitamins and fibre.

4 Crab Sticks with Sweet Chilli Dip

Maybe not as posh as king prawns, but crab sticks still pack a lot of taste into a small amount of calories! Like most seafood, crab is high in protein and low in fat, as well as boasting a host of other vitamins and minerals. The sweet chilli dip will help to counter sweet cravings, while giving your metabolism a quick boot at the same time.

½ **Small Avocado with Lemon and 1 tbsp Prawns**

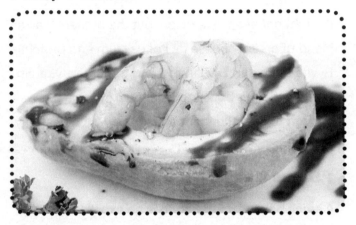

Avocado is often rejected as a diet 'don't' because it contains high levels of fat. But it's the type of plant fat (polyunsaturated) that is essential for proper cell structure and functioning, rather than the animal type that sticks to your thighs. Avocados are high in vitamin E (which improves skin health) too, so served with protein-rich prawns, this snack packs all the punches.

2 Tuna Sushi

Two pieces of tuna nigri makes a great snack, because it's filling and nutritious — protein and omega fats from the fish, carbs, fibre and vitamins from the rice. If you can, opt for brown rice instead of white: it provides slow release energy and contains higher levels of B vitamins.

1 oz Smoked Salmon and 1 tsp Cream Cheese

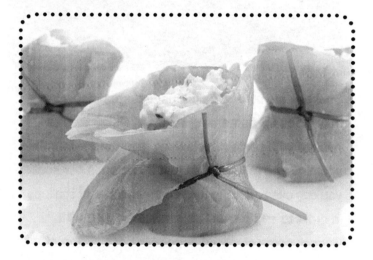

Tucking into a plate of smoked salmon can feel like a real treat, but not one that is particularly calorific, even when teamed with its ultimate partner, cream cheese. Just think — all that protein, calcium and omega goodness, and none of the guilt? Be sure to opt for low fat cream cheese.

5 Large Scallops

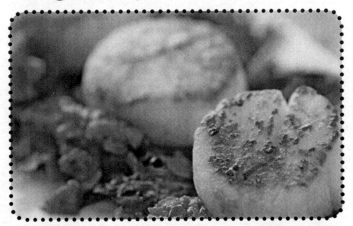

Scallops are meaty, delicious and suprisingly low in calories for something so tasty, PLUS they're packed with protein, selenium, and other essential vitamins and minerals. At just 20 calories per scallop you can even afford to reduce the number of scallops in order to add a small side salad dressed with vinegar, some steamed vegetables or a dollop of light mayonnaise.

6 Oysters with Lemon and Tabasco

What could be more decadent than six fresh oysters with lemon and Tobasco? Not only are oysters extremely tasty, they're also packed with protein and complexion-clearing selenium, as well as a host of other immune system and energy boosting vitamins and minerals.

Grilled, Skinned Chicken Breast with 1 tsp Light Mayo

A diet tip to remember: the stronger and more powerful your muscles are, the more calories you will burn — and faster. To do this, you need to feed your muscles with an adequate amount of protein (15-20g every day), as well as working them out from time to time. A grilled chicken breast is a great snack food option, because it's low in fat and high in protein.

1.5 oz Turkey Meat with Stewed Cranberries

Like chicken breast, turkey is also high in muscle-strengthening protein and low in fat. But dark turkey meat is particularly nutritious, because it contains twice the amount of beauty-boosting zinc and riboflavin as the white part of the meat. Both these minerals are essential for maintaining a healthy immune system, so teamed with antioxidant-rich cranberries, you have a pretty unbeatable partnership.

½ Apple Sliced and Dipped in Peanut Butter

Yes, peanut butter is scarily high in calories, but in small amounts it can be a delicious snack booster! Here, you can combine its fibre and protein-rich nutrients with a satisfying, antioxidant-packed slice of apple to form this surprisingly tasty snack. Opt for natural, rather than salty, peanut butter.

A 227g Jar of Gherkins

A whole jar! Really? Put it this way, pickles are so low in calories that if you're a big gherkin fan you can pretty much eat as many as you like for a snack! These pickled cucumbers are mineral-rich and contain no fat whatsoever. They do contain high levels of salt though, which can be harmful to the body when consumed in large quantities, so don't eat too many jars at once!

2 Cups of Popped Corn

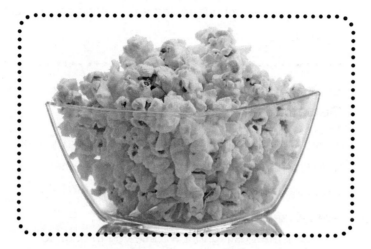

Popcorn is fast becoming one of the most popular diet snacks around, thanks to it being extremely low in fat and calories (and mainly full of air). Just make sure you don't cancel all this out by adding butter, toffee, or other calorific substances. Opt instead for cinnamon (a powerful metabolism booster) or a small amount of salt, instead.

½ Cup of Frozen Yoghurt

Frozen yoghurt is the perfect decadent yet low calorie snack for those looking to lose weight. Like all calcium and protein rich foods, it's filling, as well as being just sweet enough to satisfy your after-dinner dessert craving without tipping your calorie count over the edge.

10 Plain Baked Tortilla Chips and Salsa

Go for baked, wholemeal tortilla chips rather than the fried type and you have yourself a snack winner. Combine them with a dollop of spicy tomato salsa, and you've got the perfect blend of energy and metabolism-boosting that will see you through to your next meal , yet feel deliciously decadent.

A Frozen Banana

Just by freezing, a regular banana is transformed into a sweet, cold and very delicious ice lolly. Bananas are also rich in fibre, potassium (a mineral essential for proper brain and nerve function) B vitamins and complex carbohydrates, too, making it a good all-round snack, particularly for providing an energy boost before exercise.

2 tbsp of Pumpkin Seeds

It might not seem like much, but two spoons of pumpkins seeds are all you need for a quick, protein-rich pick-me-up in between meals. Pumpkin seeds are high in vitamin E, too, so are a good all-round beautifying ingredient to sink your teeth into.

¼ Cup of Edamame Beans

This means a ¼ cup out of their shells, not in them! Edamame beans — or soybeans — are extremely low in fat, and boast high levels of muscle-strength-ening protein and fibre. Soya is also thought to have anti-aging and collagen-boosting properties too, so good for your skin and your tummy!

20 Strawberries

Strawberries are a great snack option because they are low in calories, high in fruit sugars and rich in fibre. They are also a potent source of antioxidants, and contain naturally-occurring plant chemicals which can boost the production of collagen — the substance that gives skin its elasticity.

3 Kiwi Fruit

Kiwi fruits are particularly satisfying, because they are high in fibre and natural fruit sugars, regulating blood sugar levels and keeping us feeling fuller for longer. They are also rich sources of vitamin C, which helps to promote a healthy immune system. You don't have to eat all 3, and could even mix and match with berries and melon chunks to create a delicious fruit salad!

Cup of Blueberries

Blueberries are often heralded as a diet hero, and not without good reason. They are low in calories, high in fibre, and even higher in antioxidants, which battle harmful toxins in the body and help to prevent illness. Blueberries are also thought to contain powerful anti-aging nutrients, earning them their so-called 'super food' status.

30 Cherries

If you're a real desk snacker while you work, you could do worse things than replace that bag of sweets or crisps with a bowl of delicious fresh cherries. Cherries are low in calories, and high in antioxidants, making them a satisfying snack that are low in calories and bursting with sweet goodness.

1 Melon (Watermelon or Honey Dew)

Yes, you read it right — one **WHOLE** melon! It's hard to believe, because they are huge, that a whole melon is so low in calories. But delicious melons, particularly watermelons and honey dew, are so diet-friendly because they are mostly made up of water and fruit sugars, which are filling and prevent sweet cravings.

150g Natural Low-Fat Yoghurt

Foods rich in calcium, like yoghurt, are great at promoting a natural feeling of fullness and well-being. Going for a low-fat option reduces your calorie intake, while protein levels stay just as high. Just beware of yoghurts that contain added sugars to counter the fat reduction, as it could up the calorie count considerably.

Carrot Sticks with 2 tbsp Hummus

Hummus is another food that is often excluded from diet plans because it is relatively high in calories. But the chickpea and sesame paste is worth every calorie — it's rich in 'good' polyunsaturated vegetable fats, as well as protein and antioxidants. And when eaten with fresh carrots it's an even better snack food.

Corn on the Cob

Corn on the cob is a vitamin- and fibre-rich food type that is low in calories, so long as you steer clear from the temptation to cover the whole thing in butter, you'll be fine! Opt for a low fat vegetable spread or olive oil instead.

2 Wheat Crackers with Peanut Butter

Peanut butter is ok in small amounts, as it is high in 'good fats' and protein, which make you feel fuller, especially when enjoyed on a fibre-rich wholemeal cracker or two.

6 Squares of Dark Chocolate

Dark chocolate is lower in saturated animal fats than milk or white chocolate, and higher in metabolism-boosting caffeine, too. It's also packed with toxin-fighting antioxidants. So snap off six small squares, sit back, and enjoy.

Six Dried Apricots

Dried apricots are delicious and easy to carry around, as well as keeping you feeling full and satisfied in between meal times. This is because they contain particularly high levels of fibre, as well as complex fruit sugars, which regulate blood sugar levels. They are a good source of vitamin E, too, which is essential for skin, hair and nail health.

2 Mini Boxes of Raisins

Now you obviously don't need to eat both boxes, but at just 50 calories per mini box, replacing your usual bag of chocolate treats with a box of sweet, tasty raisins is a great choice your waistline will thank you for!

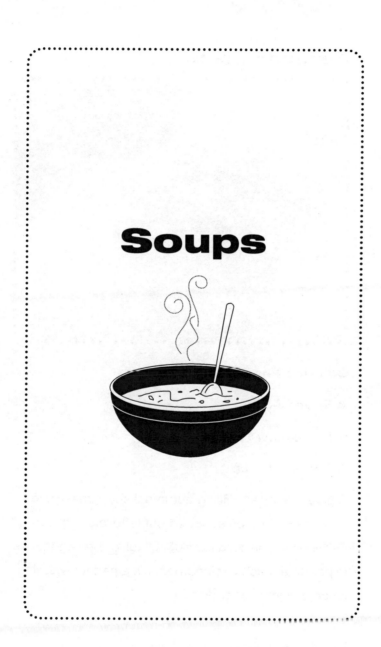

Soups

Pumpkin Soup

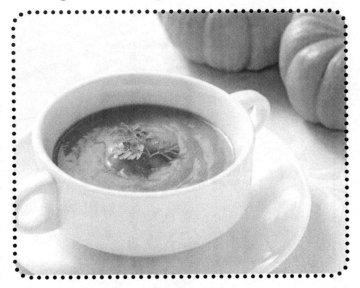

Calories Per Serving 178

✳ *Serves 4-6*

✳ *Preparation 15 mins*

✳ *Cooking 1 hour*

A great hearty and filling autumnal soup, make use of those Halloween scooped out leftovers with this delicious recipe. Healthy but still full of flavour, thanks in part to a touch of cinnamon, it's a perfect warming lunch or light supper dish.

Ingredients

250g pumpkin flesh

1 onion

750ml chicken stock

2 carrots

Pinch of cinnamon

Salt & pepper, to taste

Method

Cut the pumpkin into little squares. Peel the onion and carrots and cut them into small slices.

Place all vegetables with the chicken stock into a saucepan and a pinch of cinnamon. Then simmer until the pumpkin flesh is soft and smooth (this will take about half an hour). Pour into a blender — you may have to do a batch at a time and never fill the blender more than half full — and whizz until all the chunks are gone and you have a smooth, soup like consistency. Return to the pot to heat. Add salt and pepper to taste.

Sweet Potato and Carrot Soup

Calories Per Serving 164

٭ *Serves 4-6*

٭ *Preparation 15 mins*

٭ *Cooking 1 hour*

Another great smooth autumnal soup that feels creamy and decadent but is low in calories and packed full of flavour and goodness.

Ingredients

250g sweet potatoes, peeled and diced
3 carrots, peeled and diced
1 onion, chopped
750ml chicken stock
Salt & pepper, to taste

Method

Add the onions to a large non-stick saucepan with a little oil and, over a low-medium heat "sweat" until they are soft but remain clear. Don't let them brown.

Add the chopped sweet potato and carrot and pour in ¾ of the chicken stock. Allow to simmer for 30 minutes or until the vegetables feel soft when you insert a knife.

Pour into a blender — you may have to do a batch at a time and never fill the blender more than half full — and whizz until all the chunks are gone and you have a smooth, soup like consistency. Return to the pot to heat. Add more chicken stock to thin the mixture if it is too thick, and add salt and pepper to taste.

Roasted Tomato Soup

Calories Per Serving 176

✳ *Serves 4*

✳ *Preparation 30 mins*

✳ *Cooking 30 mins*

In summer, if you have a glut of homegrown tomatoes, this soup could be made in batches and frozen in perfect portions, ready for each Fast day!

Ingredients

750g ripe tomatoes, quartered

1 onion, chopped

1 large carrot, quartered lengthways

2 cloves garlic, chopped

1 tsp olive oil

1 x 400g can of chopped tomatoes

1.25l chicken or vegetable stock

1 tbsp chopped fresh basil, to garnish

Extra virgin olive oil, to garnish

Method

Preheat the oven to 180°C. Line a roasting tray with baking parchment.

Spread the tomatoes, onions, carrot and garlic cloves onto a baking tray. Roast for 20-30 minutes, or until caramelised.

Transfer to a large saucepan and add the tinned tomatoes and stock. Bring to the boil, reduce the heat and simmer for 30 minutes. Remove from the heat and allow to cool a little. Purée the soup in batches in a blender or with a hand-held blender. Season to taste with salt and black pepper. Serve hot, garnished with chopped basil.

Garden Vegetable Soup

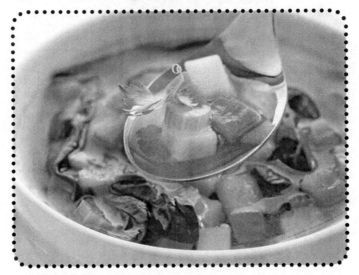

Calories Per Serving 120

✳ *Serves 4*

✳ *Preparation 10 mins*

✳ *Cooking 30 mins*

If you are vegetarian you can use vegetable stock instead of chicken stock, and also substitute any vegetable you don't like for a vegetable you do like.

Ingredients

½ tsp basil

¼ tsp oregano

¼ tsp salt

500ml chicken or vegetable stock

250g green beans, chopped

250g turnip or swede, diced

6 carrots, chopped

2 cloves minced garlic

1 onion, chopped

1 tbsp tomato paste

Method

In a large saucepan sprayed with nonstick cooking spray, sauté the carrot, onion, and garlic over low heat until softened, about 5 minutes.

Add the stock plus all the remaining ingredients and bring to a boil. Lower the heat and simmer, covered, about 15 minutes or until beans, carrots and swede are all tender. Add any salt and pepper to taste.

Chicken Noodle Soup

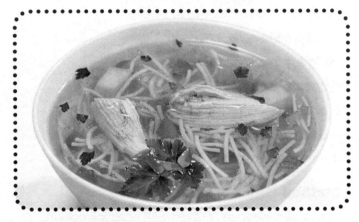

Calories Per Serving 200

✳ *Serves: 4*

✳ *Preparation Time: 5 mins*

✳ *Cooking Time: 15 mins*

Chicken Noodle soup is a tasty, filling meal in a bowl and the perfect way to use up any leftover chicken from the Sunday roast! You can either use home-made chicken stock, or if you prefer the fast and easy approach simply use shop-bought stock cubes/melts.

Ingredients

2 litres of chicken stock

Shredded chicken, as much as you have, around 3 handfuls is ideal

5 carrots, peeled and roughly chopped

3 celery stalks, chopped into bite-sized pieces

2 onions, medium-sized, diced

1 clove of garlic, crushed

Bay leaf, parsley and thyme — or a shop-bought sachet of bouquet-garni

Tsp salt

Tsp ground pepper or crushed peppercorns

30g butter, unsalted

2 nests of dried egg noodles, or 1 x 400g bag of fresh egg noodles

1 spring onion, chopped, to garnish

Method

Add the butter to a large pot and melt over a medium heat. Add diced onions and chopped celery, and cook until onion turns clear. Be careful not to brown or burn the onion or celery. Add the chicken stock, carrots, herbs and seasonings and simmer on a low heat until the carrot chunks are tender. Add the shredded chicken and noodles, cook for a further 5 minutes on a low simmer. Divide into bowls. Serve with some chopped spring onion to garnish.

Light Lunches

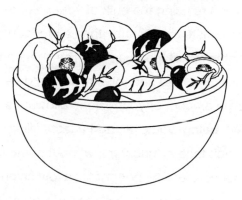

Light Lunches

Many people on the 5:2 opt to skip lunch and save the majority of their calories for their evening meal — but if you've skipped breakfast, or just find it impossible to get through a busy, working day without eating something, then a light lunch is the ideal option.

Unless you're using the bulk of your calories at lunchtime instead of dinner, then a big fat baguette is probably out of the question. The sheer amount of calories in bread and rolls mean you'd be using up a large amount of your calorie allowance on the roll itself, before you even add a tasty filling. Instead, if you can't face a lunchtime without some sort of carbohydrate, why not got for a low calorie wholemeal wrap or pitta bread filled with something lean and tasty — low in calories but high in taste and satisfaction. Crispbreads and granary bread, in moderation are also a good choice.

Most of these recipes can be easily made at work, or prepared in advance and taken with you, and they are all under 200 calories, leaving you plenty left over for dinner tonight!

Wraps

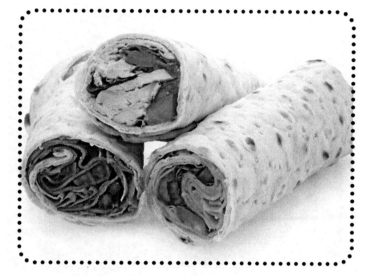

A typical wholemeal wrap contains around 130 calories, so you can then choose your fillings depending on how many more calories you have to play with.

Great lean and healthy choices include:

Wafer thin ham, prawns, turkey slices, chicken, lean roast beef. Avoid calorie-laden dressings like mayonnaise and instead go for a light balsamic salad dressing, or a couple of tablespoons of the delicious tomato salsa (recipe below).

Tomato Salsa

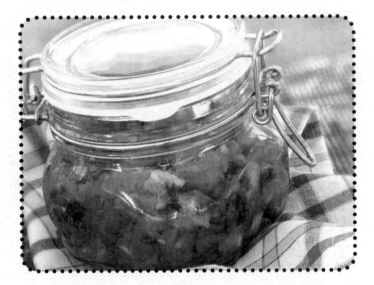

This delicious tomato salsa can be made in bulk, stored in the fridge and used to liven up all sorts of dishes. It's perfect to add to wraps, pittas, pour over chicken breasts, or just used as a lovely, tasty and fresh side accompaniment to pretty much anything. And, the calories involved in a couple of spoonfuls are tiny! You can choose lemon or lime juice, and even add in chopped cucumber for a bit of variety.

Ingredients

3 medium sized tomatoes
½ a medium red onion

The juice of one lemon or lime

Olive oil, drizzle

Handful of chopped coriander/cilantro

Salt and pepper to season

Method

Dice the tomatoes and red onion, squeeze the lemon or lime juice into mixture. Finely chop the coriander and add, together with a drizzle of olive oil, to the bowl. Add a seasoning of salt and pepper. Transfer to a freezer bag, jar or plastic tub. Shake to mix all the ingredients. Store in the fridge, and it should last for up to a week.

Chicken Kebabs with Peppers Salad

Calories Per Serving 210

Cut a chicken breast into 1" chunks and thread onto wooden kebab skewers. Grill, then served with a chopped yellow and red peppers or small side salad. Drizzle with the juice of 1 lemon for added flavour and moisture.

Chicken Breast with Tomato Salsa

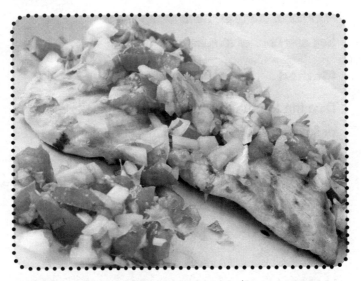

Calories Per Serving 185

Chicken is always a great low-calorie, high protein option that keeps you feeling fuller, longer. Liven up a grilled chicken breast with a few spoonfuls of the delicious tomato salsa, and if desired served with a side salad. A perfect, easy, tasty lunchtime filler.

2 Crispbreads with Cream Cheese and Smoked Salmon

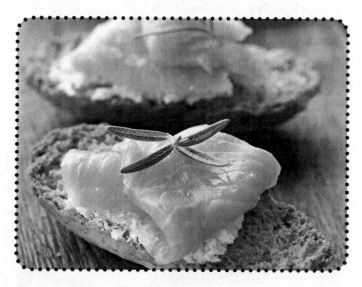

Calories Per Serving 170

When you need taste AND crunch for lunch, crispbreads are an obvious choice. Many shop-bought
crispbreads are only around 35 calories each, leaving
you plenty of calories for a tasty topping. Top each
crispbread with 1 slice of smoked salmon and 1 tsp
of low calorie cream cheese.

Beans on Toast

Calories Per Serving 175

Top one slice of granary toast, with 50g of baked beans — the ultimate comfort food !

Mozarella and Tomato Salad

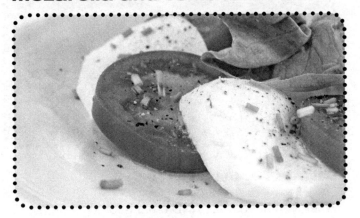

Calories Per Serving 185

Feeling Italian? Take 3 slices of low-fat mozzarella and one large beefsteak tomato (or 2 regular tomatoes). Slice and lay on a small plate, drizzle with a mixture of olive oil and balsamic vinegar and top with chopped, fresh basil. A taste sensation at under 200 calories!

Flatbread pizza

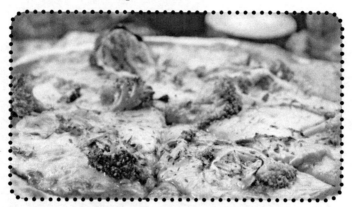

Calories Per Serving 220

This is one of my favourite lunches, and it also works well as an evening meal, accompanied by a side salad. With a wholemeal wrap coming in at just 130 calories, I figured it made the perfect low-calorie "pizza base". Spread 2 tablespoons of chopped tomatoes, or shop-bought pizza sauce, and top with 30g of low-calorie grated mozzarella. Finish with some chopped, fresh tomatoes, and you have a huge, delicious low-cal "pizza" at a fraction of the calories of a deep dish!

If you're having this for a main meal, or have extra calories to use, add a couple of slices of ham, or sliced mushrooms, to make it extra special.

Chilli Prawn Pitta Pockets

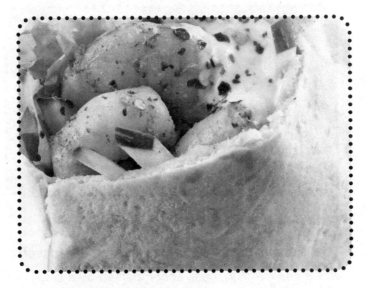

Calories Per Serving 180

Like wraps, at around 120 calories, wholemeal pitta bread is a great lunchtime choice. Split open your pitta bread and fill ¾ with a green salad, dressed with a low-calorie balsamic salad dressing.

Sprinkle 8 large prawns with chilli powder and/or paprika, grill or cook in a pain for 2 mins each side (or until cooked). Drizzle with lemon juice and add to the pitta bread. Simply delicious!

1-egg Pepper and Onion Omelette

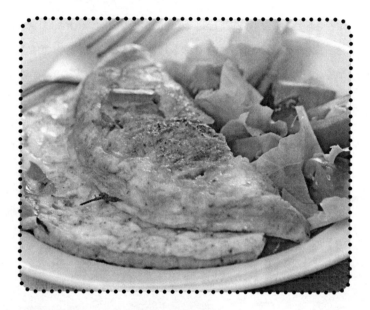

Calories Per Serving 145

Add a tablespoon each of diced onion and diced red pepper to a non-stick frying pan (or one that has been sprayed with low-calorie cooking spray). Cook on a medium heat until the onions are cooked but clear and the peppers have softened.

Meanwhile – break a large egg into a bowl and add a tablespoon of skimmed milk. Season with a little salt and pepper, and if you have any chopped, fresh herbs (coriander, basil etc) feel free to add these for extra flavour.

Whisk briskly to get lots of air into the mixture, then add the cooked onion and pepper to the bowl. Spray your pan again, return to the heat and pour the contents of the bowl into the hot pan. Do not stir! Let the mixture start to cook, and start gently lifting the omelette around the sides, nudging any runny parts over the egde to ensure that all the egg mixture is cooked. When the eggs are no longer runny in the centre and the omelette has set, flip one half over the other and slide onto your plate. Serve with a small green salad.

Meals

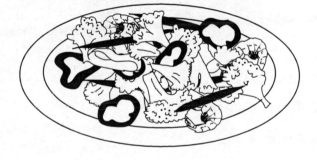

Cajun Cod

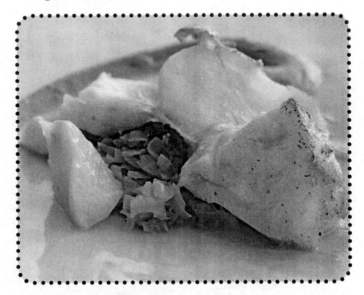

Calories Per Serving 185

❊ *Serves 4*

❊ *Preparation 5 mins*

❊ *Cooking 15-20 mins*

The mildness of cod takes well to bold flavourings such as Dijon mustard and Cajun seasoning. Lemon juice, added after cooking, brightens the flavour. If you can't find Cajun seasoning in the supermarket, make your own: Combine 1 tablespoon paprika with

1 teaspoon each of salt, onion powder, garlic powder, dried oregano, ground red pepper, and black pepper.

Ingredients

2 tsp olive oil

2 tsp Dijon mustard

½ tsp salt

½ tsp Cajun seasoning blend

4 cod fillets (about 1 inch thick)

Cooking spray

1 tbsp fresh lemon juice

Method

Preheat oven to 200°C/gas mark 6 /400°F.

Combine the olive oil, mustard, Cajun seasoning and salt; brush evenly over the code pieces.

Place fish on a foil-lined baking sheet coated with cooking spray. Bake for 17 minutes or until the fish flakes easily when tested with a fork. Drizzle the lemon juice evenly over fish, and garnish with parsley, if desired.

Pesto Fish Kebabs

Calories Per Serving 195

* *Serves 4*

* *Preparation 10 mins*

* *Cooking 8-10 mins*

You can make this fresh, colourful and tasty 20-minute meal with just 4 simple ingredients. This recipe uses halibut but you can easily substitute any white, meaty fish like cod or monkfish. A shop bought jar of pesto is ideal for this.

Ingredients

700g halibut, cut into 1-inch chunks
1 large red pepper, cut into 1-inch chunks
3 tbsp basil pesto
2 tbsp white wine vinegar
½ tsp salt
Cooking spray
Kebab skewers — wooden or metal

Method

Preheat oven to 200°C/gas mark 6 /400°F.

Mix together the pesto and white wine vinegar in a small bowl.

Place the fish chunks and peppers in a shallow dish. Drizzle the pesto and vinegar mixture over the fish mixture and toss to coat. Let fish mixture stand 5 minutes to absorb the flavours.

Thread the fish and pepper chunks alternately onto each of 4 (12-inch) skewers; sprinkle evenly with salt. Place the skewers on a flat baking tray coated with cooking spray. Bake in the oven for 8 minutes or until the fish chunks are cooked (but not dried out), turning once.

Tomato Tart

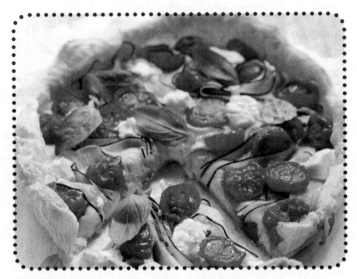

Calories Per Serving (⅛ tart) 275

✳ *Serves 8*

✳ *Preparation 15 mins*

✳ *Cooking 40 mins*

This delicious tart, served with a side serving of sweet cherry tomatoes and a handful of salad, makes a delicious summer meal.

Ingredients

200g ready-made shortcrust pastry/pie dough

Cooking spray

70g fontina cheese, shredded

½ cup pitted kalamata olives, chopped

⅓ cup sliced shallots

3 large heirloom/beefsteak tomatoes, seeded and cut into ½ -inch-thick slices

3 tablespoons plain / all-purpose flour

1 tbsp thyme

1 tsp salt

½ tsp pepper
300ml semi skimmed milk

1½ tbsp grated Parmigiano-Reggiano
3 large eggs
2 tablespoons fresh basil leaves
1 cup cherry tomatoes, quartered
1 bag of rocket/arugula
Drizzle of balsamic vinegar

Method

Preheat oven to 180°C/gas mark 4/350°F

Roll out the dough to a 12-inch circle; press into a 9-inch deep-dish tart or springform pan coated with cooking spray. Sprinkle with the cheese , olives, and shallots. Arrange half of the tomato slices over the shallots. Combine the flour and thyme; sprinkle over tomatoes. Top with remaining tomato slices; sprinkle with ¾ teaspoon salt and pepper.

Next combine the milk, Parmigiano-Reggiano, and eggs and pour into pan over the tomato and shallot mixture.

Bake in the oven for 40 minutes or until set, then let stand 10 minutes. Top with fresh basil leaves.

Toss the rocket and cherry tomatoes, then drizzle with the balsamic vinegar to create a delicious side salad. Slice the tart and serve with the salad.

Mexican Salsa Chicken

Calories Per Serving 210

* *Serves 4*

* *Preparation 10 mins*

* *Cooking 25 mins*

For this easy chicken recipe you can use your favourite shop bought tomato-based salsa and taco seasoning mix to create a filling and low calorie taste of Mexico!

Ingredients

450g skinless, boneless chicken breasts, cut into bite-sized chunks

2 tsp mexican taco seasoning

Cooking spray

230g tub of tomato salsa

70g shredded reduced-fat cheddar cheese

¼ cup fat-free sour cream

Sliced green chilies

2 tbsp sliced ripe olives

Method

Preheat oven to 200°C/gas mark 6 /400°F.

Combine the chicken chunks and seasoning in a

medium bowl, tossing to coat. Heat a large nonstick pan, coated with cooking spray over medium-high heat. Add the chicken; cook for 4 minutes or until browned, stirring occasionally. Arrange chicken in an 8-inch square baking dish coated with cooking spray; top with salsa, cheese, and chilies. Bake for 8 minutes or until the chicken is cooked thoroughly and the cheese is melted. Top each serving with 1 tablespoon sour cream and a sprinkling of olives.

Sweet and Spicy Prawns with Rice Noodles

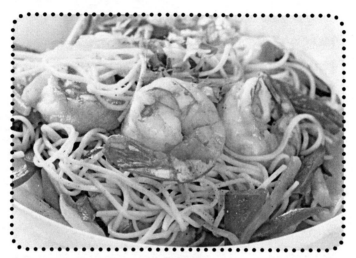

Calories Per Serving 280

✻ *Serves 2*

✻ *Preparation 30 mins*

✻ *Cooking 5-10 mins*

If you're craving an oriental take-away, try this fresh, tasty low calorie option instead!

Ingredients

1 tbsp rice vinegar

2½ tsp honey

1 tbsp sambal oelek (available from oriental

97

supermarkets or aisle)

1 tbsp lower-sodium soy sauce

240g peeled and deveined medium shrimp/prawns

120g, or 2 nests of uncooked flat rice noodles

(pad thai noodles)

1 tbsp peanut oil

2 tbsp chopped unsalted cashews

1 tbsp thinly sliced garlic

1 tbsp chopped red chilli

2 tsp chopped peeled fresh ginger

1 red and 1 yellow pepper, sliced

¾ cup matchstick-cut carrots

¼ tsp salt

¾ cup of mange tout

¾ cup fresh bean sprouts

2 sprigs fresh coriander/cilantro, chopped

Method

Combine the first 4 ingredients in a medium bowl, stirring well with a whisk. Add prawns to vinegar mixture; toss to coat. Cover and refrigerate for 30 minutes.

Meanwhile, cook the noodles according to the package directions, then drain. Rinse with cold water.

Heat a large skillet or wok over medium-high heat.

Add oil to pan; swirl to coat. Add cashews, garlic, ginger, and chilli to the pan.

Stir-fry everything for 1 minute or until the garlic begins to brown.

Remove this mixture from pan with a slotted spoon, and set aside in a bowl.

Increase heat to high, and add the red and yellow peppers, carrot, and salt to the pan, and stir-fry for 2 minutes.

Add the prawns and vinegar mixture to the pan (do not drain). Stir-fry for 2 minutes.

Next, stir in the noodles and mange tout; cook for 1 minute, tossing to coat evenly. Now return the cashew mixture to the pan. Add the bean sprouts; cook for 1 minute or until thoroughly heated, tossing frequently.

Serve in a cereal sized bow, sprinkle with fresh coriander garnish.

Chilli Con Carne and Tacos

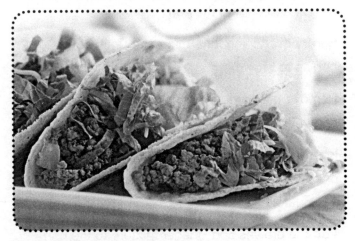

Calories Per Serving 300

✳ *Serves: 4*

✳ *Preparation Time: 5 mins*

✳ *Cooking Time: 25 mins*

Chilli Con Carne is a big favourite in my family, so when the kids are enjoying theirs with a mound of white rice, I discovered taco shells — a great low-calorie way to enjoy chilli. I like the *Old El Paso* ones from the supermarket, which are just 67 calories per shell. By adding lots of salad to each shell before I put in the chilli, it makes for a crunchy, spicy delicious meal.

Ingredients

Drizzle of olive oil OR non-fat cooking spray

450g / 1lb extra lean beef mince

1 large onion, chopped

1 red pepper, chopped

2 garlic cloves, crushed (or 1 teaspoon very lazy garlic)

2 x 400g tins of chopped tomatoes

1 x 200g tin of red kidney beans (drained and rinsed well)

1 red chilli, de-seeded and finely chopped (or 1 tsp very lazy chilli)

1 tsp tomato puree

1 tsp each of cumin, coriander, paprika and chilli powder

Method

Use the olive oil or non-fat spray to oil a large saucepan, place over a medium heat and add the mince, onion, chopped pepper and garlic. Stir regularly until all the mince is browned. Add the chopped chilli and the various herbs to the mince and stir thoroughly. Now add the chopped tomatoes, tomato puree and kidney beans. Stir gently and cook over a medium heat for around 15-20 mins. Taste to see if chilli is spicy enough — you can now add any additional chilli or seasoning to suit your personal taste.

Serve with 2 shop-bought taco shells (or more, depending on your calorie allowance) with salad.

Cumin-Coriander Sirloin Steak

Calories Per Serving 245

✻ *Serves 2*

✻ *Preparation 5 mins*

✻ *Cooking 20 mins*

The combination of cumin, coriander, and ground red pepper create a tasty rub for the beef, and the brown sugar caramelises beautifully. Heating the cast-iron skillet results in a flavourful seared crust on the steak without having to first brown the meat on the stovetop.

Ingredients

Cooking spray

1 tbsp brown sugar

½ tsp salt

½ tsp ground cumin

½ tsp ground coriander seeds

¼ tsp ground red pepper

2 sirloin steaks (about 1¼ inches thick), trimmed

Method

Preheat oven to 220°C/gas mark 7/425°F.

Coat an 8-inch cast-iron skillet with cooking spray. Place the pan in the pre-heated oven for 5 minutes.

Combine the brown sugar, salt, cumin, coriander seeds and pepper, and rub over both sides of steak. Place the steak in the preheated pan.

Bake for 7 minutes on each side or until desired degree of doneness. Let it stand 5 minutes. Cut steak diagonally across grain into thin slices.

Pan-Fried Sole with Cucumber and Tomato Salsa

Calories Per Serving 230

* *Serves 4*

* *Preparation 10 mins*

* *Cooking 3 mins*

This simple pan-fried fish is brightened with a mild but colorful fresh salsa. Any variety of sole or flounder will work in this recipe — try lemon sole or butter sole.

Ingredients

2 cups cherry tomatoes, roughly chopped

¾ cup cucumber, finely chopped

⅓ cup yellow pepper, chopped

3 tbsp chopped fresh basil

2 tbsp capers

1½ tbsp finely chopped shallots

1 tsp balsamic vinegar

2 tsp grated lemon rind

1 tsp salt

¼ tsp freshly ground black pepper

1 tablespoon olive oil

4 (6 oz) sole fillets, skinned

Method

To make the salsa, combine the first 8 ingredients in a bowl, then add in ½ teaspoon of the salt and teaspoon of the black pepper.

Heat the olive oil in a large nonstick pan over medium-high heat. Sprinkle the fish with the remaining salt and black pepper. Add the fish to the pan, and cook 1½ minutes on each side or until the fish flakes easily when tested with a fork. Spoon over the salsa to serve.

Grilled Chicken Caesar Salad

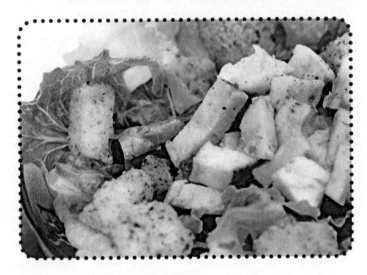

Calories Per Serving 295

✳ *Serves 4*

✳ *Preparation 5 mins*

✳ *Cooking 10 mins*

This crunchy and tasty salad mimics the flavour of a typical Caesar salad, but in a vinaigrette form, so with much less fat and calories.

Ingredients

Small baguette, cut into ½-inch cubes (about 2 cups)

Cooking spray

2 skinless, boneless chicken breasts, cut into strips

½ tsp black pepper

2 tbsp white wine vinegar

2 tbsp olive oil

1 tsp minced garlic

1 tsp Dijon mustard

½ tsp anchovy paste

6 cups chopped romaine lettuce

Click to see savings

2 cups chopped radicchio lettuce

100g grated fresh Parmesan

Method

Preheat oven to 180°C/gas mark 4/350°F

Spread the bread cubes in a single layer on a baking sheet. Bake for 10 minutes or until lightly toasted.

Heat a non-stick frying pan or skillet over a high heat. Coat the pan with cooking spray. Sprinkle the chicken with ¼ teaspoon pepper. Add the chicken to the pan, and cook for 3½ minutes on each side or until done. Remove from pan; let stand 5 minutes. Cut the chicken into slices.

For the dressing: Combine the remaining ¼ teaspoon pepper, vinegar, olive oil, minced garlic, mustard and anchovy paste in a large bowl, stirring with a whisk. Add all lettuce to the bowl and toss well to coat.

Divide the lettuce and chicken evenly among each of 4 plates.

Top each serving with ½ a cup of the croutons and 1 tablespoon of the grated parmesan.

Breaded Chicken Parmesan and Salad

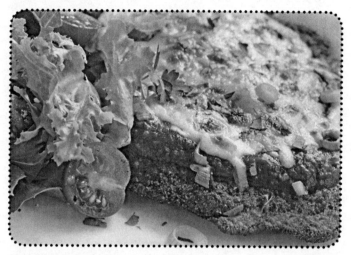

Calories Per Serving 300

* Serves 2

* Preparation 5 mins

* Cooking 10 mins

This dish has the same great taste of the Italian favourite, but this one is good for you!

Ingredients

2 skinless, boneless chicken breasts

1 tbsp grated Parmesan cheese

¼ cup Italian-style bread crumbs

1 tsp garlic powder

1 tbsp onions, dried

Crushed red peppers if desired

1-2 tbsp olive oil

1 jar of marinara/tomato sauce

Method

Preheat oven to 200°C/gas mark 6/400°F.

Cut the chicken breast horizontally (fillet it) so you will end up with two thin pieces.

Rub each piece with olive oil.

Mix all the dry ingredients together, then toss each chicken piece with the crumb mixture until well covered.

Bake in the oven for about 20 minutes or until chicken is cook through.

Meanwhile, heat tomato sauce in a saucepan. Pour over chicken to serve. Serve with a tossed lettuce, onion and tomato salad drizzled with balsamic vinegar.

James' Favourite Jamaican Jerk Chicken

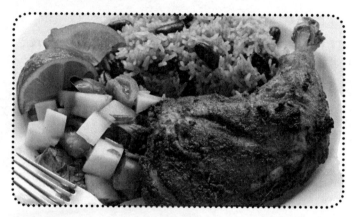

Calories Per Serving 250

* Serves: 4

* Preparation Time: 2.5 hours (allows for marinade)

* Cooking Time: 30-35 mins

Jerk chicken is one of my absolute favourite chicken dishes — it's so packed with flavour yet low in calories and can be eaten on its own, or served with rice, salad or a tasty salsa, depending what your calorie total allows.

Ingredients

4 large chicken legs, or 8 thighs

1 large onion, chopped

2 tablespoons olive oil

For the Marinade:

1 tbsp each of : All spice, brown sugar

*1 tsp each of: Ground black pepper, salt, thyme, nut-
meg , cinnamon*

3 crushed garlic cloves (or 2 tsp of lazy garlic)

*1 red chilli, de-seeded and finely chopped (or 1 tsp very
lazy chilli)*

*2 fresh limes — squeeze the juice form each to add to
marinade*

Method

Place all the marinade ingredients into a large freezer
bag , seal and shake well to mix into a paste. Add
the onion and chicken, seal the bag and shake well
to ensure all the chicken is coated. Refrigerate for at
least 2 hours, overnight is even better, and turn the
bag occasionally to coat all the chicken pieces.

Preheat oven to 200°C / gas mark 6 / 400°F

Bake chicken in the oven in a deep dish, covered
with foil, for 30-35 minutes (checking chicken is
cooked all the way through before eating). Serve with
salsa, salad or rice depending on how many calories
you wish the meal to be.

Beef Stew

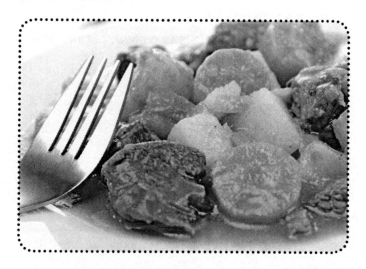

Calories Per Serving 400

✳ *Serves: 4*

✳ *Preparation Time: 15mins*

✳ *Cooking Time: 3 hours*

During the cold winter months, nothing beats a hearty, warming stew. Even on the 5:2 we can still enjoy our comfort dishes, and by using lean meat and lots of vegetables, this heart-warming dish comes in at 400 calories for a good-sized serving. Slow-cooked for 3 hours, the meat will just melt in the mouth.

Ingredients

Olive oil & cooking spray

900g / 2lbs of lean beef stewing steak, cut into bite-sized chunks

2 large onions, chopped

4 large baking potatoes (or 8-10 regular potatoes) peeled and cut into bite-sized chunks

4 large, or 6 small carrots, chopped

4 crushed garlic cloves (or 2 tsp of lazy garlic)

1 x 400g tin of chopped tomatoes

80g (1/3 cup) plain flour

250 ml (1 cup) red wine, preferably dry but any leftover red will do

250ml (1 cup) of beef stock – made from stock cubes or melts is fine

1 bay leaf

Thyme (1 tbsp chopped fresh thyme, or 1 tsp dried thyme)

Salt & pepper to season

Method

Preheat oven to 150°C / gas mark 2 / 300°F

Heat a large casserole dish over a medium heat on the hob, and coat well with a low-fat cooking spray. Add the chopped onion and garlic and sauté until the onion is clear and soft. Scrape this mixture into a large bowl, and re-coat the pan again before adding half of your beef chunks to the pan. Brown the meat for 5 minutes, again over a medium heat, tossing to ensure it is browned on all sides. Move this meat into the bowl with the onions and garlic, and repeat the browning process with the remainder of the beef chunks, then transfer these to the bowl too.

Pour the red wine into the pan and allow it to reach a boil, stirring well. Return the beef, onion, garlic mixture to the pan. Pour in the beef stock, plus a cup of water. Add in the carrot, bay leaf, herbs and seasoning and pour in the tin of chopped tomatoes. Stir well to combine all the ingredients.

Turn off the hob, add the lid to the casserole dish, and transfer into the oven. Cook for 1 ½ hours, then add in the potatoes. Also, in a cup, combine ¼ cup of water with the flour and mix until smooth. Add this into the casserole and stir in well to help thicken the stew. Cover dish again and return it to the oven. Cook for another 1 ½ hours or until the beef chunks, potato and carrot pieces are tender. Fish out and discard the bay leaf, then your Beef Stew is ready to serve!

Peanut-Crusted Chicken with Pineapple Salsa

Calories Per Serving 225

✳ *Serves 4*

✳ *Preparation 10 mins*

✳ *Cooking 10 mins*

If it's in season, you can use fresh pineapple in this recipe, otherwise substitute with tinned chunks from the supermarket; chop into half-inch pieces for the salsa. Serve with steamed broccoli for a delicious low calorie dinner.

Ingredients

1 cup chopped fresh pineapple or pineapple chunks

2 tbsp chopped fresh coriander/cilantro

1 tbsp finely chopped red onion

1/3 cup unsalted, dry-roasted peanuts

1 slice of white bread

1/2 tsp salt

1/8 tsp black pepper

4 medium sized chicken breasts

1 1/2 tsp sunflower oil

Cooking spray

Method

To make the salsa, combine the pineapple, coriander and red onion in a small bowl, tossing well.

Combine the peanuts and slice of bread in a food processor and process until finely chopped. Sprinkle salt and pepper evenly over the chicken, then coat each breast with the breadcrumb mixture.

Heat the sunflower oil in a large nonstick pan over a medium heat. Add chicken to pan; cook 4 minutes on each side or until the breast is cooked through and not pink in the middle. Serve the chicken with the pineapple salsa mixture and fresh, steamed broccoli.

Turkey Meatballs in a Tomato Sauce

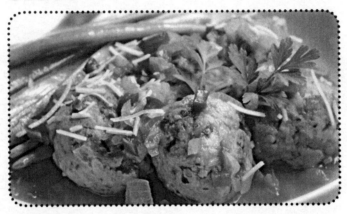

Calories Per Serving (6 meatballs) 280

✻ *Serves: 4*

✻ *Preparation Time: 15 mins*

✻ *Cooking Time: 20 mins*

Meatballs are another big hit with my friends and family, and by replacing beef mince with turkey mince, you can pack a lot of flavour in for a lot less calories.

Ingredients

350g/12oz fresh turkey mince

1 x 400g tin of chopped tomatoes

1 large onion,chopped

2 stalks of celery, finely chopped

3 crushed garlic cloves (or 3 tsp lazy garlic)

2 tbsp mixed herbs (chopped fresh, or dried)

25g/1oz breadcrumbs

3 tbsp Parmesan cheese, grated

Salt and freshly ground black pepper to season

1 medium egg, beaten

1 tbsp olive oil

Method

Combine the turkey mince with the herbs, bread-crumbs, parmesan, salt, pepper and half of the garlic. Add the beaten egg and mix well with your hands until the mixture starts to bind together. Roll into 24 small balls – each about the size of a walnut.

Heat the olive oil in a large non-stick frying pan and add the turkey balls. Stir regularly to ensure the meatballs are browned all over. Once browned, move the turkey balls into a bowl.

Now add the onion and remaining garlic to the pan, and sauté until the onion is soft and clear, and not browned.

Return the turkey meatballs to the pan, pour in the tinned tomatoes and reduce the heat. Allow the mixture to summer, stirring occasionally, for 10-12 minutes. Remove one meatball, cut in half to ensure it is cooked all the way through. If so, your meatballs are ready to serve. A green side salad is the perfect low-calorie accompaniment to this meaty Italian meal.

Individual Cottage Pies

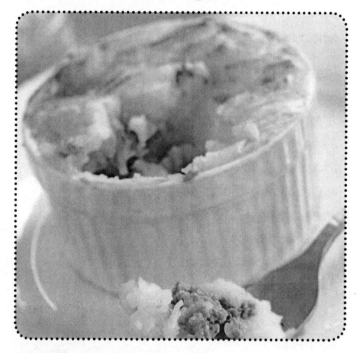

Calories Per Serving 180

٭ *Serves: 8*

٭ *Preparation Time: 5 mins*

٭ *Cooking Time: 30 mins*

Another family favourite but this time, by using mini ramekins to help with portion control, you can get your Cottage Pie fix whenever you feel like it.

This recipe makes 8, so you can pop each individual portion in the freezer, and even take them to work to reheat for lunch!

Ingredients

450g/1lb lean ground beef mince

1 large onion, chopped finely

3 large carrots, chopped

3 crushed garlic cloves (or 2 tsp lazy garlic)

450g/1lb bag of frozen peas

1 tsp rosemary

1 tsp mixed herbs

salt and pepper to season

240ml /1 cup of beef stock

3 cups or one shop-bought pack of mashed potatoes

Method:

Preheat oven to 200°C / gas mark 6 / 400°F

Coat a large frying pan with low-calorie cooking spray and add the chopped carrots, onion and garlic. Cook until the onion is soft but clear and the carrots have started to soften.

Add the mince, rosemary and herbs and cook until the mince is browned throughout. Pour in the beef stock and add the frozen peas, and cook the whole mixture until the peas have thawed.

Divide the mince mixture between 8 ramekins, and top with mashed potato. My wife likes to use an icing piping bag and nozzle for this part to make our pies look nice and fancy!

Bake in the oven for 20 minutes. Then serve with plenty of vegetables — carrots, broccoli, green beans and cauliflower work well.

Italian Chicken Casserole

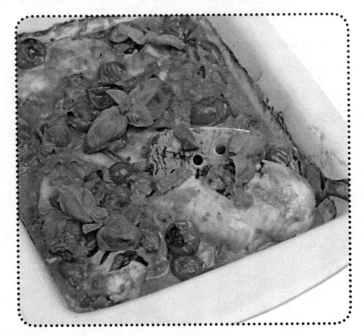

Calories Per Serving 250

✳ *Serves: 4*

✳ *Preparation Time: 15mins*

✳ *Cooking Time: 30-40 mins*

This tasty tomato-based chicken casserole feels indulgent and decadent, but when served with a fresh salad comes in at just 250 calories (plus your choice of salad dressing).

Ingredients

4 large chicken legs, or 8 thighs

2 large onions, chopped

2 tablespoons olive oil

3 crushed garlic cloves (or 2 tsp lazy garlic)

1 x 400g tin of chopped tomatoes

600g/21oz ripe tomatoes

2 tbsp tomato puree

1 bay leaf

1 tsp dried rosemary (or chopped, fresh)

Salt & pepper to season

Handful of fresh basil leaves

Method

Preheat oven to 200°C / gas mark 6 / 400°F

Place a large, non-stick pan pan over a high heat on the hob, and add the olive oil. Season each chicken piece, then add to the pan, browning each chicken piece thoroughly on each side. You may need to do this in 2 batches, depending on the size of your pan. Put the browned chicken to one side.

Reduce the heat to medium and add the onions and garlic to the pan, and cook the onion until soft and clear. Return the chicken pieces to the pan, and add all remaining items — tomatoes, chopped tomatoes, pure and herbs (everything except the fresh basil leaves) to the pan. Stir well. Transfer to a baking dish and cover with foil. Bake in the oven for 30-40 minutes, until each chicken piece is cooked thoroughly. Garnish with fresh basil leaves and serve hot, with a fresh green salad.

Chicken Breasts stuffed with Spinach and Cheese

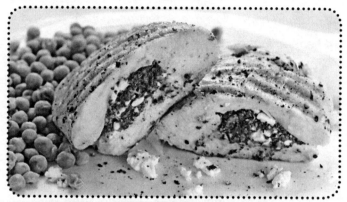

Calories Per Serving 195

* *Serves: 4*

* *Preparation Time: 15mins*

* *Cooking Time: 25-30 mins*

This cheesy stuffed chicken feels rich, creamy and decadent, yet is surprisingly low in calories. If you don't have *Light Philadelphia* in the fridge you can substitute any other low fat soft/cream cheese — we like to use *Light Dairylea* or *Laughing Cow* triangles too — one per chicken breast ,spread on first before the spinach mixture is added. If you have extra calories to play with, you can wrap each breast in parma ham, lean bacon or pancetta for extra flavour

127

Ingredients

4 chicken breasts (boneless, skin removed)

2 crushed garlic cloves (or 2 tsp lazy garlic)

4 heaped tablespoons Philadelphia or other

low-fat soft cheese

1 x 200g bag of spinach

Salt & pepper to season

1 tbsp olive oil

Method

Preheat oven to 200°C / gas mark 6 / 400°F

Steam or microwave the spinach for 1 minute so it starts to wilt. Mix together the soft cheese and garlic in a bowl, add the wilted spinach and mix it all together. Add a seasoning of salt and pepper.

Make a slit across the middle of each chicken breast big enough to stuff in the spinach and cheese mixture, before securing each breast closed with a wooden toothpick.

Place in a foil wrap and put on a baking tray. Bake for 25-30 minutes or until the chicken is cooked through. Delicious!

I do hope you've enjoyed the recipes in this book, and they go some way towards helping you with the success of your 5:2 diet journey!

Good luck, stay healthy, be happy, and if the 5:2 works for you — pass the message on!

If you have found this book helpful, it would be greatly appreciated if you would take a moment to post a review on amazon. Reviews can help others decide if a book might be helpful for them, and sharing your 5:2 story can help inspire others to give it a go !

Best Wishes, and Good Luck!

James Drummond

Lightning Source UK Ltd.
Milton Keynes UK
UKOW03f0138090714

234752UK00011B/205/P